Americare
Our Moral Responsibility

Rudy Kachmann M.D.

Published by Rudy Kachmann, M.D.
www.kachmannhealth.com

Copyright © 2018 Rudy Kachmann M.D.

ISBN-10: 1986744604

EAN-13: 978-1986744607

Printed in the United States of America

Contents

Introduction	5
How to pay for it	8
Preventative care	17
Open Borders	20
A complete system	24
Healthcare card	26
Placebo and its evil twin, nocebo	29
The magic eight	33
We need a new definition for pain	36
Let's get the job done	43
Veterans	55
Overdosed America	58
Unequal treatment	64
Change is possible	67
Capitation	74
How to ensure voter turn out and save our democracy at the same time	80
Summary	82

Introduction

The purpose of this book is to propose an idea for a system of health coverage that treats everyone the same. And I believe it's important to keep this idea as simple as possible, because complexity is the enemy of success. President Trump has found that out the hard way; "I didn't know it was that complex," he said when he examined the current system. He and his party unsurprisingly failed in their efforts to write a new healthcare bill.

The enemy of everything is complexity and red tape.

I say bypass and ignore the difficulties and just move in a straight line to the vision. If it's bold enough, and inspiring enough, it will sell itself.

Health insurance should be for everyone, treating everyone the same, including members of the House and Senate and the rest of the federal government, who have great health insurance. That's one of the reasons they're not motivated to make the necessary changes. On top of that, there is always a series of middlemen who will promise to help you cut corners when the real writing of the bill occurs at the congressional level. We want to stay away from these middlemen; we just want to promote the idea of "Complete care."

A great example was a famous chancellor, Otto von Bismarck, who in the late 1800s had just united multiple independent federations to form a new country called Germany. Nevertheless, looked like he was headed for defeat in the next election because the opposition had proposed a national health plan called the Krankenkasse, along with a social security system. Bismarck was going to lose the election big-time. He solved that problem by proposing these two new social systems himself—and won the election by a landslide. Are you getting the point? The same thing happened in Taiwan. The Republicans were going to lose the election big-time, because of the proposal of national health insurance. So they proposed national health themselves and won the election. Again, are you getting the point?

If the Democrats or Republicans were to propose what I'm calling Americare, or Medicare for every American, it is my opinion the same thing would happen here. And 2018 is the ideal political year.

Building on Medicare and improving it by including vision and dental care would be a great way to appeal to voters not entrenched on either side. This of course will take some money, and I will explain where the funds will come from in the next chapter. I also think deductibles need to be lower; many people are facing deductibles at the level of thousands of dollars. You could easily capture their votes.

But the important point is that we need to focus on the big picture, fulfill the dream. Winning is the number one priority, and we need to fulfill our moral obligation to provide healthcare for everyone. Starting wars all over the world should not be a leading priority.

How to pay for it

First, I'm starting from the premise that healthcare for everyone is both a dream and a moral obligation.

We can easily micromanage this dream to death. That's what industry, pharmaceutical companies, local government, and a Congress paid off by lobbyists can do for us.

We will never beat the lobbyists. Our legislatures at the state and federal level receive millions of dollars from them.

Our only option is to outvote, outorganize, and probably outmarch them. This is an ideal political year to do this. The Republican bill has failed completely. The public is desperate and it is possible for the Democrats to take both the House and Senate in November, especially if they focus on a great issue that affects us all.

I recently attended a monthly meeting of the Allen County Division Smoke-Free Indiana. It was an excellent meeting.

There were three bills in our state legislature that would have a) reduced cigarette advertising to children, b) increased the age of smoking to 21, and c) increased the cigarette tax. The goal was to reduce the smoking rate and of course its deadly consequences.

The legislature is heavily controlled by Republicans on all sides, including the governor. All three bills were defeated. The public did not do its work, and once again industry filled the gap with their lobbying money. Is this bribery or is it the way democracy works? Either way, it did not do any of us any good.

According to the economic principle known as "elasticity of demand," if you increase the price of, or reduce access to, a product, sales will go down. Having been a neurosurgeon for 45 years, I had a front-row seat to the devastating effects of nicotine addiction, with tumors spreading to the brain, the spine, and every other part of the body. These horrible deaths are often completely avoidable. Shame on the Senate and House of Indiana.

Incidentally, Senator David Long's office in Fort Wayne is located in the Pizza Hut headquarters. The company's president and vice president were both smokers, and both died a few years ago. I personally witnessed their unfortunate deaths, and soon thereafter the deaths of their beautiful pets—a dog and a parrot. What do you think? Secondhand smoke? You would think Senator Long would stand up for any effort to address the devastation. But lack of knowledge is not the problem.

The lobbyists have the money and so they drive the discussion. On the other end, any health coverage program will cost enormous amounts of money. But we can't let that seemingly insurmountable challenge get in our way or we'll never succeed in making a national healthcare program for everyone a reality.

I'm for improving Medicare by, for example, including dental and visual care. We could also possibly include a year or two of end-of-life care. Many people have to sell a house to receive proper end-of-life care. That's not acceptable.

That's why I'm proposing this grand idea to you.

In The Healing of America, T.I. Read surveys the medical systems of a dozen countries. It's an enlightening read. You can read about England and Canada—places where the health systems are referred to as socialist by Republicans—and find that they're not as horrible as many of us assume. Anyway, even in our own country, we have the Veterans Administration, Medicare, Social Security, and a huge population on Medicaid, so you're dreaming if you think our system isn't largely socialized already. Besides, we're not talking about freebies. We're talking about a moral obligation.

In a later chapter, I'll discuss options for incorporating free market elements into the healthcare system. So I'm not proposing strict capitalism or strict socialism. Both have their merits. I'm proposing we do whatever works to ensure the healthiest outcomes for all Americans.

It is my opinion that all of us, Republicans and Democrats alike, need to look to other countries to weigh our options and arrive at the most effective solutions. Many nations use nonprofit insurance companies, which compete vigorously against each other for business.

Many Western nations also have what's known as a Value-Added Tax (VAT). It is placed on a lot of products sold on a daily basis. The consumers quickly become so accustomed to it they rarely look at it. When a country applies a VAT to healthcare, it's called a healthcare premium. The result is that you have complete healthcare coverage with very low deductibles.

Let's face it, many of us are facing deductibles in the range of thousands of dollars. Many Americans simply can't afford that, so they hesitate to go to the doctor. And then there are the costs of medications. Research suggests that patients are only taking about 50% of the medications ordered for them.

Healthcare expenses will only go up in the future, but a healthcare premium based on a VAT will be much easier to adjust than our current system of waiting for Congress, especially with their alarming new tendency to have budget shutdowns. Healthcare cannot wait. Emergencies occur daily. It's a matter of life and death.

When you add up the savings from using nonprofit insurance companies, opening the borders for more competition, regularly evaluating the usefulness of care, opening competition through the use of capitation products (which I'll discuss in a later chapter), and negotiating with foreign pharmaceutical companies, the healthcare expenditure complex looks a little bit better—contrary to the way we're doing things now, which is leading us to a huge disaster.

With a healthcare premium based on a VAT, the rich will pay more in taxes, but the costs involved will be a choice. But if you put the whole bill on the rich alone, the plan will never work. Other countries have value-added taxes, so it's nothing that unusual. Company contributions and employee healthcare costs could even be reduced while wages are increased.

The burden of rising healthcare costs faced especially by small companies would be decreased. Some companies might even relocate to the US because of our low healthcare costs. Why would a foreign company relocate to the US? They are expecting the Type II Diabetic population to double in 12 years. There are around 30 chronic illnesses associated with that disease. But a good 90% of that could be avoided through proper medical screening and wellness instruction on a regular basis, none of which is being done at the present time.

The VAT will need to increase over time because of inflation and increasing numbers of illnesses. Then again, we already have a way of paying for it. Congress is slow to act, may never act, and healthcare is just too important for that.

Remember, we must sell the vision first. But once elected, a Democratic Congress followed by a Democratic president might just get the job done. If the public does not participate, it will never happen. Step up to bat and join us in the fight. I'm not picking a generally Democratic or Republican philosophy; I'm picking one party because they might be able to do it. I just don't think the Republicans could get the job done.

Preventative care

The cost savings of preventative care could be huge. This is a conclusion I've reached after 50 years of experience in neurosurgery and wellness coaching.

Half of all medical care today it is not necessary. Let me repeat: 50% of medical care is unnecessary. Actually, it's probably a bit higher than that. I can recommend several books and documentaries full of the scientific evidence proving this point:

1. The End of Diabetes by Dr. Joel Fuhrman
2. Eat to Live by Dr. Joel Fuhrman
3. Goodbye Diabetes by Dr. West Youngberg
4. Eat Fat and Stay Thin by Dr. Mark Hyman
5. Fat Chance by Dr. Lustig
6. Secrets of the Nondiet by Dr. Kachmann
7. The 30-Day Miracle by Dr. Franklin House
8. The Fraud, the Scam of Type II Diabetes by Dr. Kachmann
9. Forks over Knives DVD
10. The China Study by Dr. Colin Campbell

I can refer you to another 20 or 30 books stating the same scientific story. They represent a real opportunity. Yet the public, Congress, and the lobbyists act like this opportunity doesn't exist. Prevention could save us probably $1 trillion.

Diabetes for instance is a problem of sugar intake. And sugar hits the brain with a shot of dopamine similar to what happens when you take drugs. Many citizens are consuming enough calories through sugar to feed an army—and they're getting sick because of it. Meanwhile, the sugar industry is getting rich.

Meanwhile, we are not testing people early enough along the path to Type II Diabetes, which comprises 30 or so chronic diseases. Dr. Mark Hyman and Dr. West Youngberg describe the correct way in their books and on their websites. I always provide a one-page handout to my patients describing that way in detail. We could diagnose most chronic illnesses 10 to 15 years before the first symptoms appear and prevent a lot of suffering—while also lowering medical costs. Most of the chronic illnesses from Type II Diabetes could be avoided. Frankly, I consider the lack off early screening to be a fraud and a scam to make a lot of money.

If people lose about 8 to 10% of their bodyweight and do some minimal exercise, eat a diet consisting of about 80% vegetables and fruit without limit, they would be very healthy.

It's simple. Yet the medical profession, government, insurance industry, and pharmaceutical companies rarely bring it up. Addressing the issue of unnecessary treatment would cut the national medical cost about 50%. Many of my patients have done that and are on no medications. Every medical visit should include a conversation about health habits. I say again, every visit.

Open Borders

Most other western nations use mainly nonprofit health insurance companies, saving about 20-30% of healthcare costs.

When you add that 25% to the 50% of treatments that are unnecessary, you start to see why healthcare costs are skyrocketing.

If we open state and national borders to competition for pharmaceuticals, medical technology, and other healthcare groups, we would probably save at least another 10-30% in healthcare costs.

If the ACA had opened at least the state borders to competition for healthcare insurance groups, patients' choices would number in the hundreds, not the one or two they have now in many states.

Let's allow even dental groups, visual care groups, and cancer treatment centers from other nations to set up clinics in this country. The savings could be huge. Recently, I had to pay $8,000 to have some teeth replaced. You might say that was cheap. I suspect if groups from different states or countries had a chance to set up business in each state, the savings might have been huge.

In Japan, they opened the market to foreign competition for MRI scans. It wasn't long before a company had invented a cheaper MRI scanner, and now you can get scanned for $150. That's free enterprise at work.

With competition between states and countries, prices will almost inevitably drop.

Germany uses hundreds of nonprofit insurance companies. In Switzerland, it's the same. All these companies are competing for customers. And the result is huge healthcare cost savings.

Enough is enough. They will say there is not enough money. But remember 50% of treatments are not needed, 20-30% profit is taken by insurance companies, probably 40% profit is taken by pharmaceutical companies, and a lot of lobbying money is wasted. The sugar and corn industries are supported by taxpayer money, and both are killing us. The idea that there is not enough money to provide complete healthcare is a complete lie. The general population appears to be okay with that; many others are not. We're trying to do something about it. Then again, we need a lot of help from dedicated people.

Many people do care, though. They know what's right and wrong. But how do you explain it when I try to get people to read free books on wellness like The End of Diabetes, Goodbye Diabetes, or The 30-Day Miracle, and 95% of them don't even bother? As a matter of fact, I brought those books to the head of public health for the state of Indiana. I also brought them to the chief diabetic educator. None of them have read these books. How do you explain that?

Now you understand why I'm saying, enough is enough.

Also, I listened to Senator Rand Paul from Kentucky speaking on the Senate floor. It was during the debate for the national budget. He's also had enough. Republicans normally vote against any increase in the federal deficit, but now when they are in power they immediately start voting in favor of increasing the deficit. How do you spell hypocrisy?

The president was right: we need to drain the swamp. But so far he's only filling it. The deficit will probably reach many trillions. And our children will have to pay for that. That is why I included a way of paying for complete healthcare.

A complete system

Most other countries use one system of medical care.

One system is clearly easier to manage, regulate, and financially sustain. It can be managed by data that's real, not what I believe or think may be the best way. Data is our future because it anchors our policies to reality and makes outcomes more predictable.

A single set of rules is necessary. What works can be proved. What does not work can be stopped. Some countries use a pricelist. Then again, if we use capitation, which I'll describe in another chapter, pricing, and capitalism, could lead the way and be even better. That discussion is something for the future. I won't digress: one-system healthcare for everyone is the first target.

One government agency will have to sort through the data and determine what are appropriate treatments. Otherwise, useless and unproven new inventions can lead the way and financially break us. It is occurring right now. Many things we providers are doing are very expensive, even though they're not scientifically proven to be effective.

The lobbyists for many food companies, the sugar industry, the technology industry, and the pharmaceutical industry are driving us into bankruptcy. They're giving our representatives so much money that I see no way of beating them at this game—unless we stand up, vote, and start marching. I do think this year is a year of opportunity that may not come back for long time.

That's why we need a board to regulate new procedures and medications. Without some centralized control, the system will implode. We are already on that road.

Health care card

For the past 15 years, France has been using what's called a "Vitale" card. In essence, it's a credit card with a gold chip that gives you a complete medical history. So you could walk into any doctor's office and once he or she downloaded it, they'd instantly know your medical past.

In my city of Fort Wayne, we don't even connect our information. All medical data between hospitals is isolated from the whole country. A card system like the one in France could be done while still protecting the health histories of the public from employers and insurance companies. Why are we so far behind?

When you leave the French doctor's office, you will know what your bill is, and within a week insurance would've paid it. Usually, insurance pays the deductible too.

As stated in my previous chapters, data is everything.

Personally, I think technology and data could have huge benefits for our medical care. I envision that when a patient walks into a provider's office, one whole wall could be the face of a computer. A patient's wristband could be activated as they walk into the room. When the provider walks in, they could say, "I want to see a lipid profile from 10 years ago, and every year since, looking for the path to diabetes." It could even be in color: blue for healthy and red as a warning signal.

The provider can then look the patient in the eye instead of being on the computer or iPad. Patients need their relationship to the provider. There is very little love between a computer and the patient. I would always say to the patient, "What's going on in your life?" This question is critical to medical care, although most of the time the provider's head is buried in the iPad or computer. That's why I say the whole wall needs to be the face of the computer, so the provider can look the patient in the eye and not be buried in the technology. I actually met with two guys who are developing such a system in Naples, Florida. So, technology can indeed bring us forward. I've said many times how important data can be. But it can also be abused.

A great deal of supposedly technological advances are really no such thing. Although there are plenty of people out there trying to sell their gizmos, we must properly evaluate every new tool.

Placebo and its evil twin, Nocebo

If I give you a red pill and you believe it might help you, there is a 70% chance that it will. Our brain produces hormones, neurotransmitters, and neuropeptides, all of which are essentially messengers that bind with receptors all over the body.

Dr. Candace Pert discovered the receptors in 1972, and she should have received that year's Nobel Prize for Medicine. She essentially proved the mind-body connection—what's going on in your mind influences what's going on in your body. Unfortunately, 40 years later, they still don't teach this in medical school.

Pert then went on to discover that the immune system produces the same triad of chemicals—hormones, neurotransmitters, and neuropeptides, like the body's own Army, Navy, and Air Force. So the relationship goes both ways; the mind influences the body, and the body influences the mind.

Our mind-body connection—with hormones, neurotransmitters, and neuropeptides—is responsible for a 50% all of our illnesses. This should be discussed extensively at every medical school. But it isn't. Just as a placebo uses the power of belief to bring about positive changes in the body, the so-called Nocebo effect is when negative beliefs lead to bad health outcomes. What this means is that a blood test—measuring levels of those three chemicals—an MRI scan, or even an angiogram could clue physicians in on problems with this mind-body nexus. And the result would be a major reduction in unnecessary treatments.

Over my decades as a neurosurgeon, I observed that MRI scans reveal something potentially amiss in almost everybody. But the issue is usually only the process of aging, and if not recognized as such, results in a lot of unnecessary surgery. Can you imagine the total potential savings to the nation's healthcare bill from orthopedic surgeons and neurosurgeons? They're doing thousands of spinal fusions every year. These doctors are good at what they do—but that doesn't mean what they're doing is necessary. In all likelihood, these patients were noceboed by doctors with an MRI scan in their hand.

We love the placebo because it can heal without costing much. Once, I had an elderly patient with severe forearm and elbow pain, and nothing seemed to work. I gave her a prescription with a label that read: Get a little dog. Guess what, it worked.

But not many people are interested in nocebos. I've talked to many deans trying to get medical schools to teach about it but they've yet to start doing so. I've even written a book, Nocebo, Placebo's Evil Twin. But few in the medical profession have bothered to read it. We could save a great deal of medical dollars and avoid unnecessary procedures and medications if providers knew about how the mind-body nexus works.

Nocebos and placebos operate by way of real neuropeptides, hormones, and neurotransmitters. Your thought process starts in the cerebral cortex and stimulates the hypothalamus, the metabolic center, sometimes called the "Wizard of Oz of your brain," to produce these chemicals that are eventually released in your body. Your monocytes, which are part of the immune system, also produce these chemicals. The mind affects the body and the body affects the mind. This has been shown by the Candace Pert's neurobiological research.

The magic eight

Keeping in mind this is a judgment-free zone, I'm going to help you see that being healthy is not complicated.

First, we'll cover the magic eight, a circle representing a culture of wellness. Second, I would like to review with you a fairly simple method of weight control and exercise. It's worked on many of my patients.

The Magic Eight

1. Self-responsibility and participating in your health is critical
2. Proper nutrition is critical; eating nutrient-dense food is the answer
3. Physical fitness represents about 25% of wellness
4. Making spirituality a part of your life can be very helpful
5. Wellness is a way of life, achievable via habit
6. The education of your genetic structure starts with birth (mother and father's health habits)

7. Learn about the mind-body-spirit connection—how you think is critical

8. Know your health risk factors, know your numbers. Yearly blood testing should begin at age 1 and results should be saved on your computer or written in a book.

Now, I'll explain another way of looking at it that's quite simple.

You have a basic metabolic rate, BMR, which represents about 30-40% of your calorie burn. This is the amount of energy your body burns up through the action of your muscles, heart, brain, etc. while you're at rest. Then you have the thermic effect of food. We only use up in metabolism about 4% of lower fat calories, which means 96% of fatty food will end up on your abdomen. Vegetables and fruit are full of fiber and water, so if you ate about 1000 calories from these types of food, only about 50% will be absorbed. The rest will exit your body in the natural way. About 30% of your calories are used up in the activities of living, your AOL. That includes things like walking the dog, but just standing up when the phone rings triples your calorie burn. Then there's the work you do, housework, sports activities, etc.

If you increase your calorie burn by about 200 calories a day, that's 20 pounds you'll lose in a year. You get my point. It's not that hard. I highly recommend increasing your AOL at work. Incidentally, there's evidence that sitting for two hours has similar effects on your body to smoking a pack of cigarettes. That's why you hear so much about standing desks and treadmill desks, etc. (If you're interested, my book Sitting Disease is available on Amazon.)

In summary, being healthy shouldn't be that difficult for you. Incidentally, eating out twice a day will not do it for you. If you like to read, get some cookbooks written by Dr. Joel Fuhrman. I recommend Quick Fix. I also like the books of Dr. Michael Gregor. If you have Type II diabetes, there's a 90% chance the chronic disease will be gone in about 30-60 days if you cook this way.

We need a new definition for pain

We've all heard about the opioid epidemic. Eighty percent of people addicted to opioids started with a physician's prescription. That to me smells of opportunity.

Our county health commissioner wants every healthcare provider to be trained to use suboxone for the opioid addicts. That will help the addicts, at least some of them. But don't forget, suboxone is also an opioid. Then again, most the time it does not cause the ecstasy and high most addicts crave, and it increases survival rates of drug addicts. Many will have to stay on the medication for the rest of their life. Addiction is a disease and for some substituting one drug for another may be the only way they can survive.

My big passion is for prevention. Remember, 80% of opiate addicts began with a provider's narcotic prescription. We Americans prescribe about 90% of the opioids in the world. Many countries have outlawed them altogether for medical treatment.

In the past 20 years, we've changed the definition of pain and started treating especially long-term pain, pain longer than 3 to 6 months, differently. Years ago, the government, CDC, FDA, veterans' administration and pain doctors like Dr. Russell Portenoy established the 0-10 rule. It's applied as follows: "What's the level of your pain on a scale of 0-10?" "I'm at nine." "Here, have some opioids."

The pharmaceutical companies have joined in and sent salespeople all over the country, which has made the epidemic of chronic pain treatment with strong opioids explode. When the patient can no longer get a prescription from their doctor, they buy heroin and fentanyl on the street, resulting in 40 to 50 thousand deaths yearly.

That resulted in my writing three books about this deadly epidemic.

The first book I wrote was The Fraud of Chronic Pain. I thought we were undergoing a national epidemic that is potentially avoidable. It is my premise that the biggest cause of the epidemic of addiction is not the drugs from Mexico and Columbia; it's medical providers' prescriptions. It was at that time that we had a huge explosion of "pain centers" all over the country. Pain specialists in these centers would start by asking, "What is the level of your pain?" The patient would say it's a 10. The pain doctor would first inject you, maybe a number times, and many made thousands of dollars. He or she would then hand you a narcotic prescription and you'd come back for a refill. Sometimes, the pain doctor would not give you a refill, but give you the injections again, making more money again, and handing you another prescription. I've visited a number these pain centers. Just sitting in the waiting room was horrific.

Seeing these patients in my office on a daily basis, I thought about alternatives. That's when I decided to open The Kachmann Mind-Body Institute in Lutheran Hospital. It is a wellness institute, where we also treat patients to avoid heart attacks, strokes, cancer, and other health issues.

The treatment of chronic pain has become a total fraud. I remember when my book came out; the whole hospital appeared to be shaking for a few days. Not one person (besides patients) said thank you. Pain centers had become nothing but cash cows.

So I designed a single-page classification scheme for acute and chronic pain. There are four classes of pain—and it couldn't be easier to understand.

1. Acute pain: heart attack, broken leg, etc.
2. Neuropathic pain: pinched nerve, neuropathy, amputation, etc.
3. Nociceptive pain: sore joint, arthritis, etc.
4. Metabolic pain: a name I suggested.

Acute pain and neuropathic pain represent only 20-25% of the pain problem. They are the only categories which should result in a prescription for opioids, and only for short periods of time. It has been amply demonstrated by research that long-term use of opioids does not work.

The other 75% of pain patients should not be given narcotics. The pain may be real, but it is based on our neurotransmitters, hormones, and neuropeptides. That's where most of the addicts come from. I call them the metabolic, or M Patients. That makes it a lot simpler, and we treat them in other ways. No narcotics. This designation alone could make a huge dent in the opioid epidemic. I gave this one-page recommendation to our county health commissioner, and although I had shown up with the coroner from Huntington County, she had no memory of the meeting when I followed up. As I already said, if we were to treat pain differently, eliminate the 0-10 pain assessment, and not give opioids to the M Patients, I think that could have a huge impact on this horrible epidemic. Can you imagine the amount of money we would save? That could be part of the new healthcare plan I'm calling Americare.

On the back of this one-page recommendation, I included some helpful guidelines:

1. Acute pain: Look for comorbid conditions including sleep apnea, heart disease, life-threatening conditions, liver disease, etc. Short-term use of morphine opioids if general health permits may be indicated and should have an end-point in mind.

2. Neuropathic pain: Should have clear evidence of nerve damage, but that alone doesn't do it. Short-term use of opioids may be necessary, but long-term use may lead to dependency and addiction. Should have 20% to 30% functional improvement or discontinue the medication. Improved function is the measure of success.

3. Nociceptive pain: Opioids should rarely be used. With no significant comorbid conditions, you may try anti-inflammatory holistic methods, physical therapy, acupuncture, and biofeedback. Medication applied to the skin and joints may also be of value. Exercise may be indicated.

4. Metabolic pain or M pain: Caused by the bumps and bruises of our life, depression, fear, anxiety, hopelessness, etc. Avoid using morphine and opioids to avoid potential habituation, dependence, and addiction. Represents at least 50% of the pain problem, with a highly overtreated population. No clear diagnosis. Avoid the pitfalls of opioid treatment. Use the functionality of the patient, which is more important than the complaint of pain in the treatment of chronic pain problems. Identifying the location of the pain will probably give you the diagnosis.

5. Chronic pain, pain lasting longer than 3 to 6 months
Proper diagnosis is critical to avoid habituation, dependency, or addiction.

Let's get the job done!!!

Running for the US Senate in a largely Republican state or for the State Senate in a Republican District may not be easy.

Then again, if you have a big dream of providing healthcare for everyone like Americare, you're putting a vision in the voters' mind and might achieve your goal.

The candidate for change has a big advantage, especially on something as big as healthcare, which reaches the mind of everyone. Many Americans have no insurance, many have poor insurance, and most of the rest have high deductibles. Vision and dental care are not paid for in any meaningful way for most people. It's on our mind every day of the week. Over 50% of my Social Security check is paid out monthly for Medicare. But remember, I still have some deductibles as well as a little reimbursement for vision and dental care. Can you imagine what that does to most people?

Scott Adams, best-selling author of The Dilbert Principle, wrote another great book, Win Bigly, which I recommend you read. I quote from it liberally. What's the point? To make a difficult sale, especially when it's very important and can help a lot of people, you may need to hypnotize your audience and give them reasons to go out and vote. You need to create passion, because many people will not get out of their chair no matter what... unfortunately.

As good as computers are today, precise polling of different districts can have an unbelievable value. That's what Donald Trump did. Why do you think in the last few days of the campaign he went to rural areas in Iowa, Wisconsin, and Minnesota?

Let's face it, some of the statements he made or tweeted might've been a bit exaggerated. What most people don't know: many of those statements had been tested in small groups.

If you're running for political office, it is natural to have some fundraisers or group discussions on specific issues like healthcare. You may need to change your language a bit depending on who you're talking to. Not many people read the newspaper and the people may not be upset about your slightly different perceptions from group to group. That's part of politics today. The group must pick up that you're addressing their problems and you behave patiently with them. You need to be biased toward big group consensus.

Trained persuaders recognize the techniques used by other persuaders in a way that the untrained do not. So going to expert advisers is critical. They'll tell you it is good to let the audience know that you are not doing it for the money but for the benefit of people like them.

I've found that true facts can be overrated. For instance, I once spoke to a health forum, and I felt I had been too loud and too passionate. I was completely wrong. The audience actually realized that I knew what I was talking about and I think they are more likely to remember what I said. Many asked for my phone number and invited me to be a speaker at their health seminars. They all knew I was not doing it for the money and that is clearly helpful. I also invited them to attend some of my other free lectures or to watch my YouTube wellness lectures for free.

Remember, humans are hardwired to reciprocate favors. If you're helping the people you're dealing with, they're more likely to go to the polls and vote for you.

Don't try bait and switch. People keep on telling me about this beautiful winter coat I'm wearing. That was a perfect bait and switch where I turned the tables on the sellers. This $250 coat was selling for $35. I couldn't believe it. So I went inside. The prettiest saleslady immediately took me to the back of the store and tried to sell me a thousand-dollar coat. I told her I will take the $35 coat and bring my wife back to show her the thousand-dollar coat. Guess what? I'm still wearing the $35 beautiful winter coat and never went back. Don't do a bait and switch on your audience. I may be sitting there and turn it around on you.

Persuasion can be effective even when the subject recognizes that technique. Keep in mind, the thing you think about the most will irrationally stay in the front of your mind. That happens to me every day. So I always ask someone in the audience what they thought of the lecture.

Sometimes you can place an intentional area of interest in the details of your message and it might attract a lot of criticism. I frankly wonder if Trump has not been doing that. He seems to hijack the TV for a week, taking a competitor right off the air. You could try speaking about your healthcare program while the other guy is constantly speaking about foreign engagements, wars for example, that most of us are not interested in. We don't want our sons dying over there.

Scott Adam says, "Facts are weaker than fiction." People have their own facts. Can you imagine listening to two people talking, one is watching CNN and the other FOX News? I've done it with one of my friends. We have never changed each other's political opinion, but we fortunately get along very well. I know of others who are completely closed-minded and I try not to speak to them.

A good general rule is that people are more influenced by visual persuasion, emotion, and repetition than they are by details and facts. Intentionally ignoring facts and logic in public is a dangerous strategy unless you are a master persuader with thick skin and an appetite for risk.

Hypnotists see the world differently. From their perspective, people are rational 90% of the time, but they know that we are almost never rational when it comes to matters of love, family, pets, policies, entertainment, and almost anything else that matters to us emotionally.

When our feelings are turned on, our sense of reason shuts off. The bad part is that we don't recognize when it is happening to us. We think we behave reasonably and rationally most of the time. Scientists have in recent years confirmed that most of our decisions are made without any appeal to the rational part of our brain. We literally make our decisions first and then create elaborate rationalizations for them after the fact.

The illusion of life is that our minds have the capacity to understand reality. But Adams reminds us we didn't evolve to understand reality. A clear view of reality wasn't necessary for our survival. Evolution cares only that you survive long enough to procreate. Each of us is, in effect, living in our own little movie that our brain has cooked up to explain our experiences. So when you're running a political campaign, keep that in mind.

Using Facebook, Instagram, and Social Media are critical, especially when the odds of you winning the race are low. You can count on your opponent using them. As Senator Dan Coats said during Senate hearings, "We are under cyber-attack from many other nations." What do you think your political opponent will be doing? You must hire a good person for that. That's how Donald Trump did it.

Creating a big vision for the public could be very helpful. And it will work even better if it fulfills a great need and seems achievable. Repeating your message many times has great value. Achieving small steps could be very helpful. Small exaggerations may not be out of place. Constant posts on social media are critical. Why you think the president is constantly on Twitter? Many people have wasted their time making fun of it, but the world is relating to it, no matter what the facts may be.

Trump is taking advantage of something called cognitive dissonance. Many people have confirmation bias. It is the human reflex to interpret any new information as being supportive of the opinions we already hold. And it doesn't matter how poorly the new information fits our existing views. We will twist our brains to make the new information feel as if it is consistent with what we know to be true. It happens in my house every day when watching one of the news programs. Many times, political positions in my house are nothing but nonsense.

Sometimes we even have mass delusions. For example, we started the war in the Middle East while almost 40,000 people die yearly from our own gun culture. The media and other organizations and politicians have done that to us. At times, we have junk science that is too often masquerading as the real thing. Our reality may not be real. We keep on hearing we need to repeal Obamacare, yet very few people really understand it enough to make their own decision. I've spoken to some congressmen with no living idea about Obamacare who want to vote it out. They don't even give you a good alternative and know very little about healthcare. I've visited our congressman in Washington, DC and know that to be true.

You have to believe yourself, or at least appear as if you do, in order to get anyone else to believe. Persuasion is strongest when the messenger is credible. Looking the audience in the eye and guessing what they are thinking can be very persuasive. I know that from my own experience of public speaking.

President Trump frequently said, "Everything that follows is true, as far as I know." After reading the book Fire and Fury, that statement worries me a bit.

A master persuader uses energy and focuses our attention through a motion-triggered visual image. Visualization speaks to the subconscious mind. That has been known for centuries, and I teach visualization techniques myself. Scott Adams, in his chapter on persuasion stack, includes the big fear, identity, smaller fears, aspirations, habit, analogies, reasoning, hypocrisy, and wordsmithing.

In my experience, visual persuasion is stronger than oral persuasion. Wordsmithing is a term invented by Scott Adams. He uses the abortion debate as an example. We all decide the debate by declaring that our definition of life must be the accurate one. You can see the point. So we can win an argument by changing the meaning of a word. We humans like to think we are creatures of reason, but we are wrong. The reality is that we make our decisions first and rationalize them later.

When doing public speaking, dress for the part, improve your physical appearance via diet, exercise, haircare, etc. Attractive people are more persuasive. Broadcast your credentials in a way that appears natural and not like bragging. People admire talent but they hate bragging. Brand yourself as a winner. Meet in the most impressive space you can control. For example, I give most of my lectures in my own auditorium, which I donated to the hospital. Set expectations ahead of time. My most common lecture is "Preventing, Stopping, and Reversing Type II Diabetes." They know what's coming. I put announcements and pictures on Facebook to pique their interest and increase the energy for the subject. I've noticed they liked my recent post of a tap dance lesson I'm taking. After all, exercise is a positive recommendation

As Scott Adams says in one of his final chapters, "Go Bigly or Go Home." If you want to win this election, you'll need to think differently. A huge vision, meeting a great need with unbelievable benefits should present the purpose of a lifetime. Good luck.

Veterans

We read about the medical care of veterans almost every day. It is also very complex.

Then again, we put a lot of money into it and we're getting a poor return. Parts of it are just great. Some of the specialized centers for limb amputations, for example, are very good. Then again, I personally examine a lot of veterans with chronic pain. Their generous medical providers essentially caused them to be addicted.

I've seen a huge number of veterans from the VA in Marion, Indiana. They handed out opioid prescriptions like they were candy. Access has been a huge problem, but they say it's improving. So I understand things are getting a bit better.

For the rest of the needed improvements, I have a very simple answer: Give the veteran the ability to choose any doctor or medical clinic in the nation, like the Mayo Clinic or Cleveland Clinic, or whatever he or she chooses. Then we can let competition clean things up. If the VA doesn't do the job, then some of the money would go to the private system. Some of that is being done already. There is a lot of resistance coming from the VA, but that resistance doesn't lead to improved service.

Also, the VA needs to write a new definition for pain. They are causing addictions and ruining the lives of many people who have served our country. That's inexcusable. These veterans have laid their lives on the line, survived combat, and then we're turning around giving them a deadly disease. Inexcusable.

About seven years ago, I read in US News about a three-star general in the US Army who had become addicted to prescription opioids following a back problem. One-third of all patients who had been treated by Army physicians became addicted to their prescription opioids. The general expressed a great desire to do something about it. I ended up meeting with him in my condominium in Naples, Florida. I even offered to join the army and help them develop a new definition for pain. I had already written three books on the topic, so I knew a lot about it. He offered to hire me, but the surgeon general of the Army disagreed. I did find out later that four big Army rehab centers in different parts of the world had stopped allowing opioid prescriptions. I know a little bit about that in detail because I met one of the rehab doctors three years later. He was working for the Army in Germany. He said that the system was developed by the same three-star general I had met. As a matter of fact, about a year later, he sent me a friendship metal.

I would give each veteran a gold card with his or her medical history embedded in a chip. So every medical provider would know what's been going on and be able to give each one the best available treatment. As already stated, I would give full choice to the veteran with no deductible, a true reward for serving our country.

Overdosed America

Commercial industry has taken over our medical knowledge.

It used to be that the government would pay for medical research. Prior to 1970, medical researchers had relatively little problem acquiring funds from the National Institutes of Health, and few medical studies where sponsored solely by drug companies. An article published in the journal Science in 1982 describes medical scientists thumbing their academic noses at industry money in the 1970s. But, as government support for medical research started to decline, scientists and universities were forced to look for alternate sources of funding for their research. The healthcare industry was more than willing to step in and lend a helping hand. Universities had no choice, and researchers' attitudes about commercial funding changed. Government funding continued to decline so that by 1990 almost two-thirds of requests for research funds from the NIH were not granted. Meanwhile, between 1977 and 1990, drug company expenditures on research and development increased six-fold, and much of the money went to support university-based research.

This shift in the sources of funding set the stage for what was to follow. Four out of five industry-sponsored clinical drug studies were still conducted by universities and academic medical centers. Academic researchers still play key roles in all phases of the research, from designing studies, to recruiting patients, to analyzing data, to writing the articles and submitting them for publication. This was not optimal for the drug and medical device companies. Research done by universities costs them more. And they quickly figured out if industry paid for the research, they could also influence the results.

Drug and biotech industries assume an ever-larger role in funding clinical trials, and they increasingly exercise the power of their growing roles in the process. Control over clinical research changed hands, quality suffered, and it all happened very quickly and with profound effects on medical practice. The roll of academic medical centers in clinical research diminished tremendously during the 1990s as the drug industry turned increasingly to new independent, for-profit medical research companies that emerged in response to commercial funding opportunities. They could play larger roles in research design, data and analysis, and even writing up the findings and submitting completed articles to journals for publication. By the year 2000, only one-third of research was being conducted by universities.

Increased reliance on private research companies allows the drug industry to kill two birds with one stone. It can now call the shots on most of the studies meant to evaluate its own products without having to accept input from academics who would ground them in traditional standards of medical science. These companies started producing drugs that were not properly tested—lots of opioid medications like OxyContin for example. They then established a new definition of pain, represented by a 0-10 scale, which resulted in huge sales numbers. How about $1 million dollars a year in sales for one opioid pain drug?

It's been said universities were seduced by industry funding, and frightened that if they didn't go along with several gag orders, the money would go to less rigorous institutions. It was a race to the ethical bottom. And it is still occurring today. I have seen this play out not only in pharmaceutical sales but also in back and joint surgery. The government will pay for new surgical interventions without clinical trials. That has been very shameful and resulted in a tremendous amount of unnecessary surgery and costs to everyone, including the government through programs like Medicaid and Medicare. We're speaking about billions of dollars.

In September 2001, an unprecedented alarm was sounded about this by the editors of 12 of the world's most influential medical journals, including The Journal of the American Medical Association, The New England Journal of Medicine, The Lancet, and The Annals of Internal Medicine.

This resulted in very little change because all the money given to our politicians by lobbyists in Washington, DC.

Commercial influence on medical research raises two kinds of concerns. First, whose drug is being studied? Those who pay the piper get to call the tune. You can design the research to match the sales program to maximize the company's profits. The questions that get answered, and thus become medical knowledge, are often not the ones that will contribute most to improving our health. We could save a lot of money if we did it right. Let's face it, changing what we eat and how much we exercise would eliminate 50-70% of chronic medical illnesses. We're speaking about $1 trillion in medical costs.

Studies repeatedly document the strong bias in commercially-sponsored research, but the medical journals seem powerless to control the scientific integrity of their own pages. The advertising in their journals pays for the publication of that journal. You get the point. But the ethical standards are horrible and the negative consequences are beyond comprehension.

When we are designing the new Americare, we need to write laws that address this issue. It will be enormously difficult because of the amount of lobbying money involved. The power of the ballot box will be necessary to save our lives. Staying on the couch will simply not do it.

Unequal treatment

You might say to yourself, "What is he talking about? Equal access and treatment options between races, culture, income levels, privileged government employees, strong unions?"

It's all those things. Remember, my position is that we have a moral obligation to treat everyone receiving healthcare the same. But you know some people think Medicaid is the best insurance. Why? Many have no deductibles; they'll even send a taxi to pick you up if you have no transportation. And it's true—matter of fact, the cost of that in the state of Indiana is higher than what they pay the doctors to treat Medicaid patients. I checked it.

You wouldn't guess who feels most offended by this. It's the middle class. Multiple family members are working, scrimping by, but can barely pay the bills, can't afford insurance, and have high deductibles. Their lives are full of fear and stress; they feed their anxieties with cigarettes, alcohol, opioids, and live in another world through excessive use of technology. I saw a family like that at my office a few years ago, two children, a mother, and a father so engrossed in their iPads and iPhones that not one of them ever looked at me during the whole 30-minute consultation, which even resulted in a necessary neck surgery because of a ruptured disc.

So there is heartburn behind free healthcare for everyone. About 25,000 New Hampshire residents paid full price for Obamacare plans last year, according to a legislative report, and their premiums increased by an average of 52% this year. This group earns more than four times the poverty level for a family of three; that's about $82,000 a year. The main problem is that deductibles went way up. It is the middle class who is getting murdered by the present healthcare system. Then again, I speak too to many well-to-do people whose deductibles are up to $10,000 a year or more. Then you might say the non-worker, the non-tax payer has no deductible.

Let's face it, some are indeed severely disabled, mentally or physically, and it has to be that way.

News stories in New Hampshire have stopped the resentment, and others facing spiking premiums have felt like giving Medicaid Platinum to those willing to pay for it and Silver for the rest. Researchers have found Medicaid recipients used healthcare more aggressively than marketplace customers, presumably because that coverage was free.

I think the only way we will ever fulfill our moral obligation and bring some fairness to the system is to have Americare.

Change is possible

You might think we are too big to change, but I don't agree with that.

I extensively reviewed the book by T. R. Reid, The Healing of America—for the third time. I agree with the author that we should take advantage all the things that work best in other countries.

That is an old Chinese saying, "To find your way in the fog, follow the tracks of the oxcart ahead of you." We are a market-driven system. New technologies I often haven't studied are introduced to medicine all the time. Most have had no clinical trials with a placebo, and the results aren't followed for fears of alternatives, etc. It seems to be working as we go. Medicare and Medicaid may even pay for using it.

Stenting for vascular disease was never properly studied by comparing the procedure to a nutrient-dense diet, a placebo, or even by following the stenting trial over a period of time.

Taiwan set up a single national insurance system. They thought the great advantage would be that you can identify more easily who is really abusing the system, or where the main costs are accruing. That allowed them to put a global budget in place. When you have a single-payer, you can say, "I'm only going to spend X percent of my GDP for health insurance," and you can control that.

Taiwan has built a system that uses private doctors and hospitals with a single government-run insurance plan to pay for them. National health insurance is not funded through general taxation; rather the money people pay to finance the health insurance fund is called a healthcare premium. They avoided the term tax. The employer and employee are required to chip in money to pay this premium. It's withheld from pay and goes directly to the government. I prefer that this premium be charged to all sales and not be the responsibility of the employee and employer. That way, you catch everyone that lives in your country and is participating in this health insurance system, which seems a lot fairer to me. The well-to-do would pay a little more because they spend more. But they also would have excellent health insurance with a small deductible. Remember, you want everyone to be treated the same.

The political party that proposed that system in Taiwan easily won the election. Does that tell you something? Their government insurance allows patients to pick doctors, so providers ended up competing fiercely for customers. I would be concerned that that could result in a lot of unnecessary treatment. The doctors in Taiwan work very hard, because they have to use volume to make up for the low fees. I'm not sure if that is actually good.

I reviewed the English system as well. It's hard to get an elective operation done, so the line is long. But this cuts down on unnecessary surgery big-time. Patients don't get a bill there. Also, I must admit they have absolutely big-time, huge-time, wellness programs. They give you phone numbers you can call anytime, there are reminders to get preventative testing done, and efforts to teach you what a proper lifestyle is—I can go on, and I repeat they are big-time into prevention. Matter of fact, as a family doctor, you're making a very good living because you're rewarded mainly from the British health service for preventative treatment. It has always been my opinion that the main job of a family physician should be teaching prevention to patients. It will be best for the patient—plus it keeps the cost way down.

Taiwan's new health insurance system may be the most efficient in the world. They spend only 2% of the cost for administration versus 20-30% spent by US insurance companies. That's a huge savings that we could clearly take advantage of by designing Americare for all. We spend about 17% of our GDP on healthcare versus 6% in Taiwan.

The plans succeeded in Taiwan because of a confluence of several conditions. The primary force for change was a strong national feeling about the moral question. There was a strong public demand for universal health insurance like the one going on in this country right now. Secondly, they had an entrenched political party with a parliamentary majority that was challenged by a rising opposition party that had openly embraced universal health insurance. We have a similar situation here. They also had sustained economic growth like we have. The similarities are obvious; this opportunity may not come again for a long time.

Switzerland, a nation of 8 million people, who speak four official languages, has also had the need for healthcare reform.

This population likes everyone to be treated the same. Everybody gets an equal chance. That is their philosophy; they feel everyone should have equal access and basic rights. Everybody gets to vote, everybody gets a jury trial, everybody gets an old-age pension, everybody pays the same price for tickets on the national railroads. Everyone should have access to medical care.

In Switzerland, the right to medical care is not a political argument advanced by the right or left but a basic truth of modern life.

But, back in 1993, many people had no health insurance. A special task force was set up to study the national problem. They looked at the US and many other countries.

In 1994, they passed a new law called LAMal. Under this plan, health insurance was separated from employment, and families went out in the market to buy coverage. Nonprofit insurance companies were required to offer basic packages of benefits to all applicants and ensure others could not make a profit on basic health coverage. The insurance and pharmaceutical companies of course greatly objected. But in the end the insurance companies actually made more money than before. Just think, they eliminated 20-30% of healthcare costs right there. Ten years later, it was well-accepted in the country.

The people in Switzerland said, "Nobody would want to go back to the system before, when some people will opt out of the insurance." They have a system now that means everybody, rich and hopeful alike, can have the best healthcare they can provide. It's accepted, it's working, and they are happy with the changes they implemented. But the country now spends about 11% of its GDP on healthcare and that is relatively high. It is the second highest spending rate in the world.

So I'm giving you some things to think about. The system of nonprofit insurance companies, that reduces the overhead around 20%; a healthcare premium, where the funds are based on employment with some coming from government, or a healthcare premium, in essence a VAT, so everybody has to pay something. But the keys will be to have Americare offer a low deductible and the ability to see any physician or doctor in the country.

As I've said many times though, the first thing to do would be to fulfill the dream of healthcare for all, with everyone treated equally. Medicare would not be taken away, just improved. And Medicaid patients would be upgraded so that they are treated equally.

Capitation

In capitation, the unit of payment is per person. You get a certain amount of money based on the patient's age or medical condition, and you are responsible for their treatment.

For example, General Motors goes to my hospital CHS and says you are responsible for the healthcare of our 10,000 employees and we are paying you $30,000,000. GM now knows what that cost is, and CHS has to manage the healthcare for 10,000 employees and try to make a profit.

If patients aren't satisfied, then the contract can be terminated or not renewed.

What I like about this way is that it would eliminate a lot of unnecessary treatments. Personally, I think it's the only way you'll make a dent in the overtreatment problem. Remember, at least 50% of what healthcare providers do is totally unnecessary. As a matter of fact, these unnecessary treatments may injure or kill the patient. You've probably read about the number of medical errors resulting in injury or death. We're talking about a very large number.

So, under capitation, we would save money and lives.

What's nice about this system—it's capitalism at its best. People saying what you're proposing is socialized medicine would be just plain wrong.

Capitated groups could go to different associations of, say, orthopedic surgeons, cancer specialists, or neurosurgeons and have them bid for a capitated price per patient. The price of medical care would come down because of competition.

If the government fixes the price like they do in Medicaid, which is happening in Indiana for example, providers won't want to see the Medicaid patient because it doesn't pay enough to even cover the overhead in the office. For example, in my neurosurgery group, my manager said I could only see three Medicaid patients a month. We not only didn't make any money from them; we lost money. You can see the point. I personally totally ignored that corporate rule and fortunately got away with it.

I was attending a conference in Chicago and a panel of experts described how a large capitated group functioned. They were extremely data-driven and the speaker described in detail how he had complete control of the group treatment and finances. I could easily see how they would be very competitive and able to write a capitated contract. It was a beautiful example of capitalism, capitation, and yet it was also good medical treatment.

If you just pay the provider with a salary, you can see how after a while it would be natural for the provider to see fewer patients. That should be part of the healthcare of the future. Data-driven, free enterprise, and competition—I think that's the only way we could reduce costs and yet improve medical care. Providers wouldn't do as much unnecessary care because it would reduce their profit.

No insurance company needed. Unneeded surgery would decline tremendously because it's eating at the company profits.

Patient satisfaction surveys should be done regularly to check on the quality of the system. Wellness teaching would explode because it would save the company money.

The payment system could vary depending on the patient's age, sex, health status, etc. Multi-specialty clinics could bid for part of the contract. A capitated model could be part of their business. They may use other systems for other patients, for example. Again, free enterprise and competition in the end would help us develop the best models and improve medical care.

Providers could be separate from hospitals or a hospital system could own the whole product.

Capitation payment would transfer to the best providers of medical care. It would discourage unnecessary treatment because they would lose the money. Wellness teaching would increase because it would increase their profits. I think it may be the only way we can stop them from overdoing it. They would do fewer procedures and prescribe less medication as part of the contract.

Just think, if the provider had to pay for the prescription, do you think we would be having 80-year-old patients on 15 different drugs, like I see commonly, most of which are unnecessary and causing a lot of complications?

Numerous studies have shown incentives under capitation have a great effect on provider behavior. Again, data will drive the system.

Clearly, it will work better if it's a completely closed system including hospitals and providers. One could keep track of it a lot easier.

No payment system is perfect. All countries have financial problems with medical care. Yet most Western nations have complete healthcare. Here in America, though, we pay the most and get the least.

Researchers have found that fee-for-service systems increase costs the most. If you go to a provider who does a certain procedure, what do you think he is most likely to do? Wellness teaching is rare. Ninety percent of vascular disease, for example, can be avoided by proper nutrition. How many cardiologists do you think are explaining that to the patient? Most cardiologists have never read the books of Dr. Caldwell Esseltyne of the Cleveland Clinic, who has written extensively on this issue. Watch the DVD Forks over Knives; it will tell you the whole story.

How to ensure voter turnout and save our democracy at the same time

During the last national presidential election, 43% of the people did not vote.

That, in the long run, could destroy our democracy. Don't believe me? Argentina for example had essentially the same democracy as a us over 100 years ago. They had poor voter turnout for decades, and eventually the military took over. That could happen to us. Did you notice the other day that our president thought it was great that the Chinese president said he will hold the office for life.

Most people don't know that a president has the power to expand the Supreme Court without need of congressional approval; it says so in the Constitution. In other words, any president could pack the Supreme Court, so we're not as safe as we might think. It is safe as long as leaders remain reasonable, but they have a legal escape clause. So we must be vigilant and appear at the polls.

Our country is becoming more polarized ethnically and racially. The Southern whites vote mainly Republican and the urban blacks democratic. They need to cooperate with each other if our nation is to survive—but they're moving farther apart.

A great antidote to this potentially scary scenario is to get them together by creating Americare. We would all be in the same boat, moving in the same direction.

All cultures, all ethnicities, all racial groups, all religious groups treated the same. It would unite us, maybe even saving our democracy if it were to become necessary in the future.

Summary

We need to be bold. We need to go and vote. We need to give financial support to good candidates. We need to show up at debates. We need to use the internet to spread the word.

Just think, the Great Health System, including Dental and Vision care, in addition to one year of end-of-life care if needed—with it, we would decrease unnecessary care, unnecessary medications, avoiding the costs and potential complications, including many deaths.

We'd all be holding hands, different religious groups, different ethnic and racial groups, young and old, it's a wonderful dream and it can be achieved. It's a moral obligation.

www.ingramcontent.com/pod-product-compliance
Lightning Source LLC
Chambersburg PA
CBHW070207230526
45471CB00002B/852